EVERYDAY PARTICIPATION

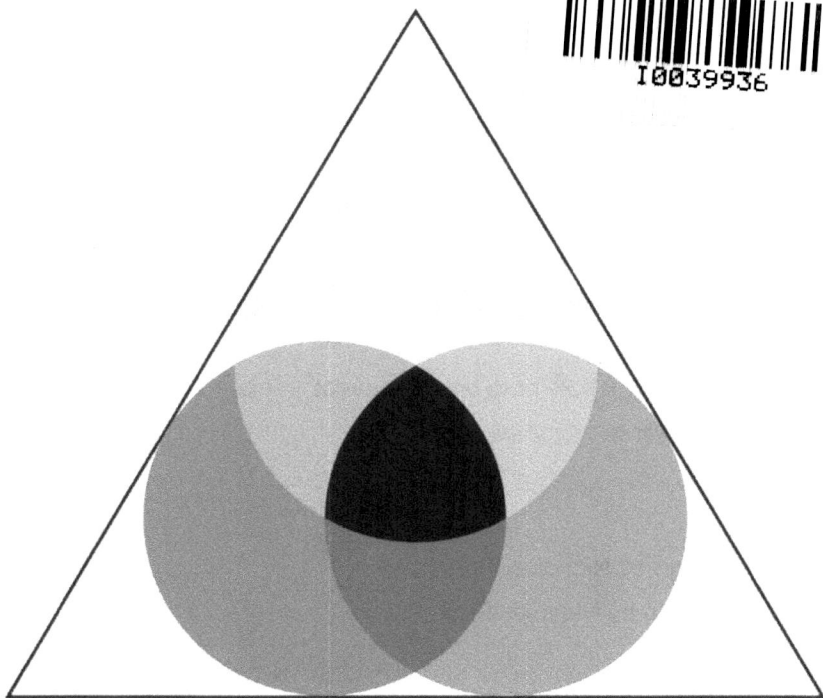

I0039936

A BLUEPRINT TO LIFELONG WELL-BEING

Nicholos Paul

For more information, or to book an event, contact:
itsowlgoodwithnick@gmail.com
www.owlgoodinvestments.com

Book design by Nicholos Paul
Cover design by Nicholos Paul

ISBN – Hardcover Book: 978-1-0689395-2-5
ISBN – Electronic Book: 978-1-0689395-1-8
ISBN – Book: 978-1-0689395-0-1

First Edition: July 2024

Dedication

To My Mom,
Your resilience has been the guiding light in my life. As a single mother raising three boys, you faced countless challenges with unwavering strength and courage. Through every battle, you remained an advocate for prioritizing health and taught me the importance of bravery, even when fear loomed large. Your wisdom and unwavering commitment to our well-being have shaped the principles I share in this book. Thank you for being the embodiment of strength and for instilling in me the values that form the foundation of "Everyday Participation."

To My Daughter,
You are the sunlight that brightens my every day. Your presence in my life has been the greatest source of inspiration, driving me to grow and strive for betterment in all aspects of my life. Your laughter and love fuel my dedication to health and well-being, not only for myself but for our family. This book is a testament to the journey of growth and health I have embarked on, inspired by your spirit. Thank you for being my constant motivation and for inspiring me to be the best version of myself for you.

To My Life Partner,
You have stood by me through every obstacle, every lesson learned, and every triumph. Your unwavering support and enduring love have been my rock, grounding me and reminding me of what truly matters. You have humbled me,

teaching me the value of respect and the importance of being a man who can be both respected and championed. Your presence in my life has been a guiding light, and your belief in me has fueled my passion to offer value to others through this book. You are my true love, and this journey would not have been possible without you by my side.

With all my love,
Nicholos Paul

A Little About Nicholos Paul

Nicholos Paul is a highly respected expert in the fields of health and wellness, celebrated for his holistic and sustainable approach to personal well-being. With a profound commitment to understanding the complexities of the human mind and body, Nicholos Paul has dedicated a part of his life to empowering individuals to achieve optimal health through practical and achievable methods.

Holding a Double Major in Kinesiology and Psychology, Nicholos Paul combines the rigorous science of physical health with the profound insights of psychological well-being. This unique blend of disciplines allows him to offer a comprehensive perspective on health that is both deeply informed and remarkably practical. His academic background laid the foundation for a lifelong journey of learning and growth, fueled by a relentless curiosity and a passion for helping others.

The cornerstone of Nicholos Paul 's philosophy is encapsulated in the acronym he coined, 'OWL'—Obsessed With Learning. This mantra has driven him to continuously expand his knowledge and refine his approach to health and wellness. By observing the intricacies of life and how various elements interact, he has developed a profound understanding of what it takes to maintain a healthy lifestyle. His passion for philosophy and keen observational skills further enriches his holistic approach, making his insights both thoughtful and deeply resonant.

Throughout his life, Nicholos Paul has maintained an exemplary standard of health, serving as a living testament to the principles he espouses. His personal rules and guidelines, which have governed his own approach to health, are meticulously laid out in his book, "Everyday Participation." These principles are not theoretical; they are proven strategies that have helped him, and countless others achieve and sustain their health goals.

People regularly seek Nicholos Paul 's advice on health matters, a testament to his credibility and the trust he has earned within his community. His ability to distill complex concepts into simple, actionable steps has made him a sought-after mentor. His approach is not about grand gestures or extreme measures but focuses on the power of small, consistent actions that seamlessly integrate into daily life.

In "**Everyday Participation**," Nicholos Paul introduces readers to a refreshing and sustainable path to health. The book is anchored by three core principles: Simplicity Focused, Achievable Focused, and Self-Aware Focused. These pillars reflect his belief that true health for the majority of the world is a marathon, not a sprint, and that success lies in the accumulation of manageable, consistent behaviors over time.

Simplicity Focused is about cutting through the noise and making health accessible by reducing complexity. **Achievable Focused** emphasizes setting realistic and attainable goals, fostering a positive cycle of success and motivation. **Self-Aware Focused** encourages a deep understanding of oneself, tailoring health practices to individual needs and preferences.

Nicholos Paul's mission is deeply personal. Having grown up with limited resources, he understands the challenges of accessing opportunities and the importance of providing others with the tools they need to succeed. He is a strong advocate of the quote, 'wisdom and knowledge shall be the stability of thy times,' believing that wisdom and knowledge are key resources for empowering oneself toward positive and proactive change. His book is more than a guide—it's a heartfelt invitation to transform one's relationship with health through simplicity, achievable goals, and self-awareness.

Nicholos Paul continues to inspire and guide readers toward a healthier, happier life. His journey is a testament to the power of knowledge, dedication, and the relentless pursuit of personal growth. Through his work, he not only shares his wisdom but also provides the resources and support necessary for others to achieve their own health and wellness goals.

Nicholos Paul lives by the principles he teaches, embodying the success and fulfillment that comes from

"Everyday Participation." Join him on this transformative journey—one small, consistent step at a time.

TABLE OF CONTENTS

INTRODUCTION

In a world where health trends and fitness fads come and go with dizzying speed, the quest for a sustainable healthy lifestyle often feels overwhelming. We are bombarded with complex diet plans, rigorous exercise routines, and an endless stream of advice that can be as contradictory as it is confusing. This book, "Everyday Participation," offers a refreshing antidote to that chaos—a practical, achievable, and deeply human approach to health and well-being.

"Everyday Participation" is not about grand gestures or extreme measures. Instead, it champions the power of small, consistent actions that seamlessly weave into the fabric of our daily lives. This approach recognizes that true health is not a sprint but a marathon, requiring a mindset and habits that can be sustained over a lifetime.

At the heart of this book are three core principles: Simplicity Focused, Achievable Focused, and Self-Aware Focused. Each of these principles is a pillar supporting the overarching concept of Everyday Participation, and together they create a robust framework for a healthy lifestyle.

Simplicity Focused is about cutting through the noise and reducing complexity in various aspects of life. Whether it's simplifying your diet to focus on whole, unprocessed foods or creating exercise routines that don't require a gym membership or special equipment, this principle makes health more accessible and manageable. The goal is to integrate these simplified elements into your daily routine effortlessly, making them a natural part of your life.

Achievable Focused emphasizes setting realistic and attainable goals. It's about making practical and sustainable changes that you can stick with rather than aiming for lofty, short-term targets that lead to burnout. By focusing on what is truly achievable, you build a foundation of habits that are not only sustainable but also empowering, fostering a positive cycle of success and motivation.

Self-Aware Focused delves into the importance of understanding oneself—mind, body, and soul. This principle encourages you to be in tune with your thoughts, emotions, physical sensations, and deeper values. Self-awareness helps you tailor your health practices to your unique needs and preferences, ensuring that the changes you make are meaningful and effective.

The synergy between these principles creates a holistic approach that is both powerful and practical. "Everyday Participation" guides you in making health a seamless part of your daily life rather than a daunting task or an unattainable ideal. By focusing on manageable, consistent behaviors, you'll find that over time these small actions lead to significant improvements in your mental, physical, and physiological well-being.

Moreover, it's important to recognize that athletes and fitness enthusiasts constitute less than 1% of the world's population. Despite this, most diet plans and exercise routines are tailored to this small, specialized group. In contrast, the remaining 99%, which includes the average person, is not striving to become professional athletes or dedicated fitness enthusiasts. Therefore, it's crucial to recognize that their approach to health and well-being should be different.

For the majority, health and fitness need to be sustainable and achievable on a daily basis. The extraordinary physical demands placed on professional athletes are not meant for lifelong engagement. This is evident from the fact that most athletes retire in their 30s, with the average career spanning less than 10 years. The rigorous training and extreme physical exertion required to perform at such high levels are simply not sustainable over a long period.

Understanding this distinction highlights the necessity for a different approach to health and wellness for the general population. Unlike athletes who push their bodies to the limit, most people benefit more from routines that promote long-term well-being. These routines should focus on consistency, moderation, and overall health rather than peak physical performance. The goal is to create habits that can be maintained throughout a lifetime, ensuring that fitness and wellness are integrated into everyday life in a practical and sustainable way.

This book is not just a guide; it's an invitation to transform your relationship with health. It's about embracing simplicity, achieving realistic goals, and cultivating a deep awareness of yourself. Through the principles and practices outlined in these pages, you will discover a sustainable path to a healthier, happier life.

"Everyday Participation" is designed to be a blueprint that can be quickly read and easily implemented into anyone's daily lives. It provides practical advice and actionable steps that you can start incorporating immediately. This book lays the foundation for a healthier lifestyle, paving the way for deeper exploration and understanding.

As you delve into this book, get ready to embark on a journey that doesn't end here. This is just the beginning. "Everyday Participation" is essentially the prequel to my next book, which will dive deeper into the research that supports what is laid out in these pages. It will also elaborate on the controversial topics that aren't widely discussed in regards to health and wellness, and thoroughly break down the actions that make the principles of Simplicity Focused, Achievable Focused, and Self-Aware Focused so successful.

EVERYDAY PARTICIPATION

The upcoming book promises to be a compelling and detailed exploration, filled with insights and evidence that will further empower you on your journey to optimal health. It will challenge conventional wisdom and provide you with the tools to navigate the complexities of health and wellness with confidence.

Welcome to "Everyday Participation." Let's begin this journey together—one small, consistent step at a time. And stay tuned for the next chapter of this exciting journey, where we will delve even deeper into the science, controversies, and practicalities of living a truly healthy and fulfilling life.

Chapter 1

EVERYDAY PARTICIPATION

Embracing the Kaizen Philosophy

In the aftermath of World War II, Japanese businesses faced the daunting task of rebuilding their economy. Amidst the ruins, a philosophy emerged that would not only transform Japan but also inspire millions worldwide: Kaizen. Derived from the Japanese words "kai" (change) and "zen" (good), Kaizen embodies the principle of continuous improvement through small, incremental changes. Popularized by Toyota, this approach became the bedrock of their production system, leading to unprecedented levels of efficiency and quality.

The power of Kaizen lies in its simplicity. Rather than pursuing radical, large-scale changes, Kaizen advocates for making small, manageable adjustments regularly. These small improvements accumulate over time, leading to significant and sustainable progress. This philosophy aligns perfectly with the principles of habit formation and sustainable health, which are central to "Everyday Participation."

The Kaizen Journey: A Story of Transformation

Consider the story of Aiko, a young professional struggling with the demands of her job. Overwhelmed and unable to maintain a healthy lifestyle, Aiko decided to adopt the Kaizen approach, making small, deliberate changes to her daily routine.

Her journey began with a single, seemingly insignificant action: placing a water bottle on her desk each morning. This small step reminded her to stay hydrated throughout the day. Encouraged by the ease and effectiveness of this change, Aiko introduced another small habit: taking a five-minute walk during her lunch break. Over time, these brief walks extended to longer periods, gradually improving her physical fitness without feeling like a burden.

Aiko's application of Kaizen didn't stop there. She began preparing simple, nutritious meals, each time making minor improvements to her recipes. These incremental changes led to healthier eating habits, which she found enjoyable and easy to sustain. The philosophy of Kaizen taught Aiko the value of patience and persistence as she witnessed the cumulative effect of her small actions transforming her life.

Integrating Kaizen into Everyday Participation

The principles of Kaizen align seamlessly with the concept of "Everyday Participation" in sustaining a healthy lifestyle. Here are some ways to integrate the Kaizen philosophy into your daily routine:

1. Start Small: Begin with tiny, manageable changes that are easy to implement. Whether it's drinking an extra glass of water or adding a short walk to your day, these small steps are the foundation of lasting habits.
2. Focus on Consistency: Emphasize regular engagement in health-promoting activities. Consistency, as highlighted by Charles Duhigg in "The Power of Habit," ensures that these actions become second nature.
3. Celebrate Incremental Progress: Acknowledge and celebrate small victories. Recognizing progress, no matter how minor, reinforces positive behavior and motivates continued improvement.
4. Adapt and Evolve: Be flexible and open to adjusting your habits. As your circumstances and needs change, adapt your routines to maintain a sustainable and healthy lifestyle.
5. Embrace Patience: Understand that meaningful change takes time. Research by Phillippa Lally shows that forming a new habit takes, on average, 66 days. Be patient and trust the process.

Aiko's Story and Everyday Participation

The story of Aiko and the Kaizen philosophy demonstrates that significant transformations are often the result of small, consistent actions. By incorporating the principles of Kaizen into "Everyday Participation," you can create a foundation for sustainable health and well-being. This approach ensures that health-promoting behaviors become an integral part of your daily life, leading to long-term improvements and a more fulfilling life. Embrace the Kaizen philosophy and begin your journey of continuous improvement today. Just like Aiko, you'll find that even the smallest steps can lead to remarkable transformations.

Key Elements of Everyday Participation

"Everyday Participation" in the context of living a healthy lifestyle refers to the consistent and habitual engagement in health-promoting behaviors that can be realistically maintained on a daily basis. This concept emphasizes the importance of integrating small, manageable actions into daily routines, ensuring they become a natural part of one's lifestyle rather than sporadic or intense efforts that are unsustainable in the long term.

Consistency:
- Definition: Regular engagement in activities that promote health, such as physical exercise, balanced nutrition, adequate sleep, and stress management.
- Importance: Consistency ensures that these behaviors become ingrained habits, which are easier to maintain over time.

Sustainability:
- Definition: Choosing realistic and achievable activities daily without causing undue stress or burnout.
- Importance: Sustainable habits are more likely to be maintained long-term, contributing to gradual and continuous health improvements.

Adaptability:
- Definition: Being flexible in approach, allowing adjustments based on individual circumstances, needs, and preferences.
- Importance: Adaptable behaviors can be maintained even when life changes, ensuring continued participation in health-promoting activities.

Incremental Progress:
- Definition: Making small, gradual changes that accumulate over time to produce significant health benefits.
- Importance: Incremental progress reduces the risk of injury or burnout and allows the body and mind to adapt steadily.

Applying Everyday Participation

Physical Activity:
- Example: Incorporating at least 30 minutes of moderate exercise, like walking, into your daily routine.

- Benefit: Regular physical activity improves cardiovascular health, strengthens muscles, and enhances mental well-being.

Nutrition:
- Example: Eating balanced, unprocessed meals with a variety of fruits, vegetables, lean proteins, and whole grains every day.
- Benefit: Consistent healthy eating habits can improve digestion, boost energy levels, and prevent chronic diseases.

Mental Health:
- Example: Practicing mindfulness or meditation for 10 minutes each day.
- Benefit: Daily mindfulness can reduce stress, improve focus, and enhance emotional regulation.

Sleep:
- Example: Establishing a regular sleep schedule with 7-9 hours of quality sleep each night.
- Benefit: Adequate sleep supports cognitive function, emotional stability, and overall physical health.

Long-Term Adaptation

By engaging in everyday participation, you create a foundation for your body and mind to gradually adapt to higher levels of health and fitness. Over time, these daily habits lead to significant improvements:

- Mental Adaptation: Regular practice of healthy behaviors enhances motivation, self-efficacy, and resilience.
- Physical Adaptation: Consistent physical activity and nutrition improve bodily functions, strength, and endurance.
- Physiological Adaptation: Long-term engagement in health-promoting activities optimizes bodily systems, such as cardiovascular, immune, and metabolic functions.

Everyday Participation is about making health a seamless part of your daily life. By focusing on manageable, consistent behaviors, you ensure that over time, these actions lead to substantial mental, physical, and physiological benefits. This approach helps preserve and enhance health, making wellness an integral and sustainable part of your lifestyle.

Chapter 2

THE TRIAD PRINCIPLES OF EVERYDAY PARTICIPATION

Simplicity Focused

"Simplicity Focused" is an approach or mindset that prioritizes reducing complexity in various aspects of life to make them more accessible, manageable, and sustainable. This concept can be applied across a wide range of domains such as concepts, methods, approaches, diets, exercise routines, and more with the ultimate goal of integrating these simplified elements seamlessly into daily life.

Essence of Simplicity

At its core, "Simplicity Focused" involves distilling complex ideas and practices down to their most essential and straightforward components. This means removing unnecessary details and focusing on the fundamental principles that can be easily understood and applied. For example, simplifying a complicated exercise routine into a basic bodyweight workout like push-ups, squats, and planks ensures consistent practice without the need for specialized equipment.

Ease of Implementation

By simplifying complex elements, the focus is on making them immediately actionable. This approach ensures that individuals can incorporate these simplified practices into their routines without extensive preparation or drastic changes, fostering a natural and effortless integration. For instance, replacing a detailed multi-step workout plan with a straightforward daily routine of a 15-minute brisk walk eliminates the barriers of needing a gym or specific equipment, making it easier to start and stick with the habit.

Sustainability and Consistency

When practices are simplified, they become easier to maintain over the long term. The goal is for these behaviors to become second nature, seamlessly blending into daily life and promoting consistency and sustainability. For example, a simple habit like a 10-minute daily stretching routine can become a sustainable part of your lifestyle compared to a complex schedule of various exercises.

Accessibility and Inclusivity

A "Simplicity Focused" approach ensures that more people can benefit from complex concepts and practices. By breaking down barriers of complexity, it makes these elements accessible to a wider audience regardless of their background or prior knowledge. For example, providing a simple, easy-to-follow exercise routine such as "10 push-ups, 10 squats, and a 30-second plank" can make fitness accessible to anyone, regardless of their experience level.

Practical Examples

Diets

Simplifying dietary plans by focusing on basic healthy eating principles like "eat more vegetables" or "avoid processed foods" rather than complex meal plans makes healthy eating more accessible.

Exercise Routines

Creating easy-to-follow exercise routines that don't require special equipment or extensive time commitments, such as a daily 10-minute bodyweight workout, promotes consistent physical activity.

Mindset and Behaviors

Encouraging simple, actionable mindfulness practices like taking deep breaths or expressing gratitude rather than in-depth meditation techniques allows for on-the-go engagement anytime, anywhere.

Explanation with Examples

Complex Concept to Simple Practice

Concept: Mindfulness meditation. Simplified Practice: Take 5 minutes each day to sit quietly and focus on your breathing.
Method: Detailed calorie counting for weight loss. Simplified Practice: Follow the principle of "eat until you're 80% full" to manage portion sizes without tracking every calorie.

Approach: Comprehensive project management systems. **Simplified Practice:** Use a simple to-do list with the top three priorities for the day. This minimizes decision fatigue and promotes productivity.

Diet: Complex Diet Plan.
Simplified Practice: Adopt a rule to include a vegetable in every meal and drink water before every meal.

Exercise Routine: Complex Exercise Routine.
Simplified Practice: An exercise that can be performed every day without machines almost anywhere and anytime, such as a daily walk for 15 minutes.

Achievable Focused

"Achievable Focused" refers to setting realistic and attainable goals, especially in the context of maintaining a healthy lifestyle.

This approach emphasizes practical and sustainable actions that can be consistently integrated into daily life rather than ambitious or extreme efforts that may be difficult to maintain.

Explanation in Context

While it's valuable to strive for growth, improvement, and success by pushing one's limits, this approach doesn't necessarily translate well to maintaining a healthy lifestyle. A healthy lifestyle should be seen as a series of essential, manageable habits rather than lofty, hard-to-reach targets.

Daily Integration

Maintaining health should consist of simple, routine actions that are easily incorporated into your daily life, much like brushing your teeth. These habits should be second nature, not requiring extraordinary effort or willpower.

Realistic Goals

Focus on goals that are within immediate reach. For instance, instead of aiming to lose a large amount of weight in a short period, the goal could be to incorporate more vegetables into your meals or to take a 30-minute walk each day. Setting realistic goals ensures that you are not overwhelmed by the enormity of the task, making it easier to stay motivated and committed.

Sustainability

Achievable Focused means setting health goals that you can sustain over the long term. This might include getting enough sleep, staying hydrated, and having regular health check-ups. These actions are manageable and can be consistently followed.

Positive Reinforcement

By setting achievable goals, you are more likely to experience success and satisfaction, which in turn reinforces healthy behaviors. This creates a positive feedback loop, encouraging you to stick with these habits.

Foundation of Well-being

These everyday actions form the foundation of your well-being. While reaching for higher achievements in other areas of life is beneficial, a healthy lifestyle is built on the consistent execution of simple, achievable habits.

Practical Examples

Nutrition: Instead of an extreme diet, aim for balanced meals with a variety of nutrients. Simple changes like adding more fruits and vegetables to your meals can make a significant impact.

Exercise: Rather than training for a marathon, start with a daily walk or a short home workout routine. Consistency in moderate exercise is more beneficial than sporadic intense workouts.

Sleep: Focus on getting a consistent amount of sleep each night rather than trying to catch up on weekends. Prioritizing regular sleep patterns helps regulate your body's internal clock.

Mental Health: Incorporate stress-relief practices like meditation or journaling into your daily routine. Regular mental health practices can prevent the build-up of stress.

Self-Aware Focused

"Self-Aware Focused" involves the conscious knowledge and understanding of one's own character, feelings, motives, desires, and overall state of being. It encompasses the ability to introspect and recognize oneself as an individual distinct from the environment and other individuals.

Mind

Psychological Awareness: This involves understanding your thoughts, emotions, and mental processes. It includes recognizing your beliefs, biases, and mental patterns.

Body

Physical Awareness: This relates to being in tune with your body's sensations, movements, and overall physical state.
Physiological Awareness: This involves understanding the internal processes and functions of your body, such as heart rate, respiration, digestion, and hormonal cycles.

Soul

Spiritual Awareness: This aspect of self-awareness relates to understanding your deeper values, purpose, and sense of connection to something greater than yourself.

Integration of Mind, Body, and Soul

Interconnectedness: Recognizing how the mind, body, and soul influence each other. For instance, understanding how stress can lead to physical ailments.

Holistic Approach: Adopting practices that nurture all aspects of your being, such as mindfulness meditation for mental clarity, physical exercise for bodily health, and spiritual practices like meditation or prayer for soul alignment.

Continuous Reflection: Engaging in regular self-reflection and mindfulness to stay aware of your internal states and how they evolve over time.

Adaptation and Growth: Using self-awareness to make informed decisions about your lifestyle, relationships, and personal development.

In Summary

Self-awareness is a multi-faceted understanding of oneself that requires conscious effort and reflection. It is the foundation for personal growth, healthy relationships, and a fulfilling life, as it enables you to live in harmony with your mind, body, and soul.

Conclusion

By embracing the principles of Simplicity Focused, Achievable Focused, and Self-Aware Focused, you can create a balanced and sustainable approach to health and wellness. This holistic method ensures that you can maintain and improve your health over the long term, leading to a more fulfilling and vibrant life.

Chapter 3

WISDOMS FOR BETTERMENT OF LIFE AND HEALTH

In Chapter 1, we delved into the philosophy of Kaizen, exploring how small, consistent actions can lead to profound and lasting changes. As we continue our journey, it's crucial to understand the broader context in which we strive to improve our health and well-being. This chapter aims to provide practical strategies grounded in the principles of Simplicity Focused, Achievable Focused, and Self-Aware Focused to help you regain control and prioritize your well-being.

Modern Mechanisms of Control

In today's society, various mechanisms subtly influence our behaviors and decisions, often without our conscious awareness. These mechanisms, ranging from advertising to social norms, shape our perceptions and habits, leading us to adopt practices that may not serve our best interests. By recognizing these influences, we can begin to reclaim autonomy over our health decisions.

Divide and Conquer

Divide and conquer is a strategy where divisions among people are fostered through political, social, or economic lines to prevent unified resistance. This tactic includes polarizing public opinion and creating echo chambers on social media, which reinforce existing beliefs and divert attention from systemic issues.

Compartmentalization and Fragmentation

Modern systems often compartmentalize tasks and information, making it difficult for individuals to see the whole picture. This creates silos that hinder communication and collaboration, making it easier for those at the top to maintain control. In both corporate and governmental contexts, such fragmentation obscures accountability and impedes meaningful change.

Deference to Authority

The tendency to not question authority, known as the white coat effect, can be exploited by institutions to shape public perception and decision-making. Milgram's experiments demonstrated this obedience to authority, which can be used to justify policies and decisions, sometimes at the expense of public well-being.

Technological Conditioning

Our reliance on digital systems often comes at the expense of critical thinking and self-reliance. Social media algorithms create filter bubbles that distort perceptions of reality, while the convenience of digital assistants and smart devices diminishes our problem-solving skills and independence.

Impact of Modern Mechanisms of Control on Self-Love

Modern mechanisms of control often program us to undervalue ourselves, subtly suggesting that we are not enough as we are. This lack of self-love can manifest in numerous ways, including poor health choices and neglect of self-care. Understanding this impact is the first step towards reclaiming our autonomy and learning to prioritize ourselves once again.

Reclaiming Autonomy through Everyday Participation

Reclaiming autonomy involves a conscious effort to make decisions that align with our true needs and values. The principles of Simplicity Focused, Achievable Focused, and Self-Aware Focused provide a framework for this journey. Each principle plays a crucial role in optimizing our ability to take control of our health and well-being.

Simplicity Focused

Simplicity Focused encourages us to strip away the unnecessary and focus on what truly matters. By simplifying our health practices, we can reduce overwhelm and create space for meaningful actions. This involves prioritizing basic, effective habits over complex routines that may be unsustainable.

- **Clarity and Focus:** By eliminating unnecessary complexities, we gain clarity on what actions truly contribute to our health. This focus enables us to make decisions that are aligned with our values and goals.
- **Reduction of Overwhelm:** Complex health routines can be daunting and lead to burnout. Simplifying these routines makes them more manageable, reducing stress and increasing our ability to maintain them over the long term.
- **Efficiency:** Simplified health practices are often more efficient, requiring less time and energy. This efficiency allows us to integrate healthy habits into our busy lives more easily.
- **Sustainability:** Simple, effective habits are easier to sustain. By focusing on foundational practices, we can build a strong, lasting foundation for our health.

Achievable Focused

Achievable Focused emphasizes setting realistic and attainable goals. This principle helps us build confidence and momentum, reinforcing the idea that consistent, small steps can lead to significant improvements. Achieving these smaller goals lays the foundation for long-term success.

- **Building Confidence:** Setting and achieving small, realistic goals boosts our confidence. Each success reinforces our belief in our ability to make positive changes, which is crucial for maintaining motivation.
- **Momentum:** Achievable goals create a sense of momentum. Each small victory propels us forward, making it easier to tackle larger challenges over time.
- **Reduced Risk of Failure:** Unrealistic goals often lead to failure, which can be demoralizing. By setting achievable goals, we minimize the risk of failure and the negative feelings associated with it.
- **Incremental Progress:** Small, consistent actions accumulate over time, leading to significant improvements. This incremental progress is sustainable and more likely to result in lasting change.

Self-Aware Focused

Self-Aware Focused is about cultivating an awareness of our own needs, motivations, and the influences around us. This awareness allows us to recognize and resist the subtle mechanisms of control that impact our decisions. It empowers us to make choices that genuinely benefit our health and well-being.

- **Recognition of Influences:** Self-awareness helps us identify external influences that may be guiding our decisions unconsciously. By recognizing these influences, we can make more informed and intentional choices.
- **Alignment with Values:** Awareness of our own needs and values ensures that our actions are aligned with what truly matters to us. This alignment makes our health practices more meaningful and motivating.
- **Emotional Regulation:** Understanding our emotions and triggers allows us to manage stress and avoid unhealthy coping mechanisms. This regulation is crucial for maintaining healthy habits.
- **Empowerment:** Self-awareness empowers us to take control of our health. By understanding our motivations and barriers, we can develop strategies that are tailored to our unique circumstances.

Practical Applications

Understanding these principles is essential, but applying them in daily life is where the real transformation happens. Here are actionable steps and examples to illustrate how you can implement these principles:

- **Identify Influences:** Reflect on the external influences affecting your health choices, such as media messages, social pressures, or habits formed in childhood.
- **Set Simple Goals:** Start with small, manageable goals. For example, instead of overhauling your entire diet, focus on incorporating one healthy meal per day.
- **Practice Self-Awareness:** Develop a routine that includes moments of reflection, such as journaling or mindfulness exercises, to increase your awareness of how you feel and what you need.
- **Consistent Actions:** Commit to small daily actions that align with your goals. Consistency, rather than intensity, is key to long-term success.

Examples and Case Studies

To illustrate these principles, let's explore some examples of individuals who have successfully applied Everyday Participation to overcome modern mechanisms of control and improve their health.

Case Study 1: Simplifying Health Practices
Jane, a busy professional, felt overwhelmed by the numerous health trends and diets she encountered. By focusing on

Simplicity Focused, she decided to adopt a simple rule: eat whole foods. This single change made her feel less stressed and more in control of her diet.

Case Study 2: Setting Achievable Goals
Mark wanted to get fit but struggled with maintaining a consistent workout routine. By embracing Achievable Focused, he started with a 10-minute daily walk. Over time, he gradually increased his activity level, leading to significant health improvements without the pressure of unrealistic goals.

Case Study 3: Cultivating Self-Awareness
Sara often felt influenced by social media trends, leading to unhealthy eating habits. She began practicing Self-Aware Focused by setting aside time each day to reflect on her feelings and motivations. This practice helped her recognize and resist the pressures to conform to unhealthy standards.

Conclusion

In this chapter, we explored how modern mechanisms of control subtly influence our health behaviors and how reclaiming autonomy through Everyday Participation can counteract these influences. By focusing on simplicity, achievability, and self-awareness, we can make consistent, manageable steps towards better health. These principles not only help us regain control but also lay the foundation for self-love and prioritization of our well-being.

As we move to the next chapter, we will build on these concepts, delving deeper into specific strategies for integrating these principles into various aspects of our daily lives. Together, we will continue to uncover practical ways to achieve sustainable, practical, and self-aware health practices.

Chapter 4

THE INTERCONNECTIONS OF EVERYDAY PARTICIPATION

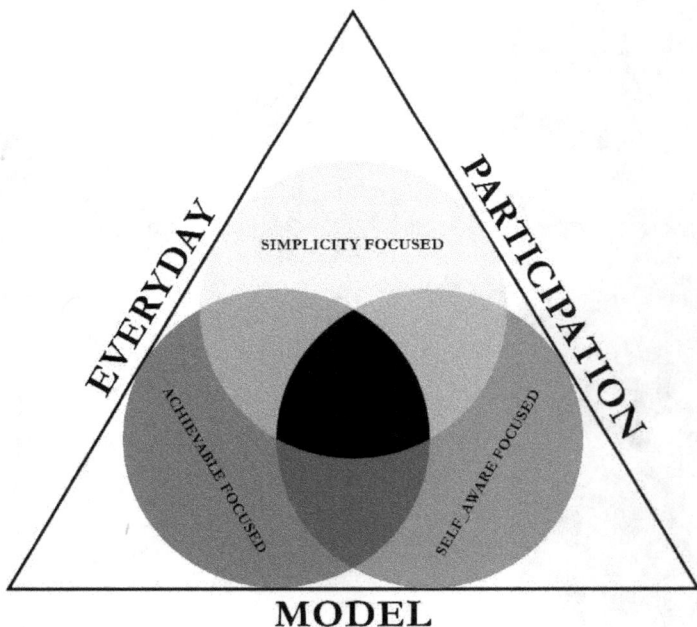

This chapter illustrates how the principles of Simplicity Focused, Achievable Focused, and Self-Aware Focused are not only interconnected but also collectively support the overarching principle of Everyday Participation. Each principle complements and enhances the others, creating a cohesive and sustainable approach to a healthy lifestyle.

Interconnections and Mutual Influences

Everyday Participation and Simplicity Focused

Interconnection: Everyday Participation benefits greatly from the simplicity of actions. When health-promoting behaviors are simplified, they are easier to integrate into daily life. For example, opting for simple whole foods over complex diet plans makes consistent healthy eating more manageable.

Influence: Simplifying tasks reduces the mental and physical burden, making it easier to engage in these behaviors daily. Thus, Simplicity Focused directly supports Everyday Participation by ensuring the tasks are not overwhelming.

Example: Imagine someone who aims to improve their overall health by eating better and exercising regularly. Initially, they attempt to follow a complex diet plan that includes specific recipes, portion sizes, and meal timings paired with an intricate workout routine involving different exercises for each day of the week. Quickly, they find this approach overwhelming and difficult to sustain, leading to frustration and inconsistency.

Recognizing the need for simplicity, they decide to simplify their diet and exercise plan. Instead of following a detailed diet plan, they choose to focus on eating whole foods: fresh fruits, vegetables, lean proteins, and whole grains. They also decide to keep their meals simple, preparing straightforward dishes like grilled chicken with a side of vegetables or a bowl of mixed salad with quinoa. This approach reduces the time and effort required for meal planning and preparation, making healthy eating more accessible and less stressful.

For their exercise routine, they opt for a daily 20-minute walk. Walking is simple, requires no special equipment, and can be done anywhere. By choosing this uncomplicated form of exercise, they eliminate the mental burden of planning varied workouts and ensure they can easily fit physical activity into their daily schedule.

Purpose-Driven Aspect: When simplifying your health practices, link them to your core values and larger life goals. This connection makes simple actions like eating whole foods or taking a daily walk more meaningful. For instance, Jane, a busy professional, not only chose to eat whole foods but also connected this choice to her goal of being a role model for her children, thereby infusing her daily actions with purpose.

Everyday Participation and Achievable Focused

Interconnection: Setting achievable goals is crucial for maintaining daily engagement in healthy behaviors. When goals are realistic, they are more likely to be met consistently.

Influence: Achievable Focused ensures that the actions taken are sustainable and do not lead to burnout or frustration. For instance, committing to a 15-minute daily walk on an incline is more sustainable than aiming for an hour-long jog four times a week. This practicality supports continuous participation.

Example: Consider an individual with a demanding job and family responsibilities who wants to improve their fitness. They initially set a goal to jog for an hour four times a week but quickly find it difficult to maintain due to time constraints and physical fatigue. Feeling discouraged, they struggle to stick to this routine.

Recognizing the need for a more achievable goal, they decide to adjust their plan. Instead of aiming for long jogs, they commit to a 15-minute brisk walk on an incline every day. This new goal fits easily into their schedule, requiring only a small portion of their day. The incline adds enough intensity to provide a good workout without causing excessive strain or requiring lengthy recovery periods.

The shorter duration and increased frequency of this activity make it easier to incorporate into their daily routine. They can walk during a lunch break, after work, or even while spending time with family. This flexibility reduces the chances of skipping workouts due to time pressures or fatigue.

As a result, they experience consistent daily participation, gradually building endurance and enjoying the benefits of regular physical activity without the risk of burnout. The success in meeting this achievable goal boosts their confidence and motivation, encouraging them to maintain and even gradually increase their fitness efforts.

Purpose-Driven Aspect: Set goals that align with your broader life purpose. This alignment ensures that each small, achievable goal contributes to your overall sense of fulfillment and life satisfaction. Mark, for example, wanted to get fit not just for physical health but to have the energy to play with his grandchildren. This purpose made his daily walks more meaningful and easier to maintain.

Everyday Participation and Self-Aware Focused

Interconnection: Self-awareness allows individuals to tailor their daily health behaviors to their specific needs and circumstances, making participation more meaningful and effective.

Influence: By understanding personal limits and preferences, one can choose health-promoting activities that are more enjoyable and sustainable. For example, recognizing that one enjoys swimming over running can lead to a more consistent exercise routine.

Example: Consider an individual who wants to include regular exercise in their daily life but finds traditional gym workouts monotonous and discouraging. Through self-awareness, they realize that they feel energized and happy when swimming. Understanding this preference, they decide to join a local swimming club and swim for 30 minutes every morning before work.

This choice not only aligns with their personal interests but also fits well into their daily schedule. They look forward to their morning swims, which serve as a refreshing start to their day. Because they enjoy swimming, they are less likely to skip their exercise sessions, leading to consistent daily participation. Furthermore, swimming provides a full-body workout, enhancing their overall fitness and well-being.

Additionally, self-awareness helps them recognize their physical limits. They might notice that after a certain duration of swimming, their muscles need a break. To avoid burnout, they balance their routine with other low-impact activities such as yoga or walking on alternate days. This approach ensures they remain active every day without overexerting themselves.

By integrating self-awareness into their daily health behaviors, they create a sustainable and enjoyable exercise routine that supports long-term participation and contributes to their overall health goals. This personalized approach makes the journey toward a healthier lifestyle both effective and fulfilling.

Purpose-Driven Aspect: Cultivate self-awareness to discover what truly matters to you and align your health practices with these deeper values. This alignment makes daily health activities not just tasks but expressions of your core identity and purpose. Sara, for instance, connected her healthy eating habits to her broader goal of achieving mental clarity and creativity in her work.

Simplicity Focused and Achievable Focused

Interconnection: Simplifying health-related goals makes them more achievable. The less complicated a goal or routine, the easier it is to stick to it.

Influence: Simplification often leads to more realistic goal-setting.

Example: Imagine someone who wants to start a fitness routine but finds traditional workout plans overwhelming. By simplifying their approach, they set a goal to walk for 30 minutes every day. This simple activity is achievable because it fits easily into their schedule, doesn't require special equipment, and can be done almost anywhere.

In addition, this person is aware that lifting heavy weights could lead to muscle soreness and require rest days, disrupting their goal of Everyday Participation. Instead, they choose to incorporate bodyweight exercises or light resistance training that can be performed daily without causing significant muscle fatigue. This ensures that they can maintain a consistent exercise routine without the need for extended recovery periods.

Simplicity Focused and Self-Aware Focused

Interconnection: Self-awareness aids in identifying which aspects of life need simplification. By understanding one's own triggers and stress points, one can simplify those areas effectively.

Influence: When individuals are aware of their tendencies towards complexity, they can consciously choose to simplify those areas, making their daily health practices more manageable and aligned with their true needs.

Example: Consider someone who finds meal planning stressful and time-consuming because they often choose elaborate recipes with many ingredients. By recognizing this stress point, they can shift towards selecting simpler recipes that require fewer ingredients and less preparation time. For instance, they might opt for meals like grilled chicken with a side of steamed vegetables and quinoa. This meal is nutritious, easy to prepare, and does not require extensive planning or cooking skills. This simplification reduces stress and makes it easier to maintain a healthy diet consistently.

By being self-aware and focusing on simplicity, individuals can make practical adjustments that align with their true needs, leading to more sustainable and enjoyable health practices.

Achievable Focused and Self-Aware Focused

Interconnection: Self-awareness informs what goals are truly achievable based on an individual's current state and capabilities.

Influence: By being aware of one's strengths and limitations, one can set more realistic goals. For example, someone aware of their limited time due to a busy schedule might set a goal to meditate for 5 minutes a day rather than 30, leading to more consistent practice.

Example: Consider a professional with a hectic work schedule who wants to incorporate meditation into their daily routine to manage stress. Initially, they set a goal to meditate for 30 minutes each day. However, they soon find it difficult to allocate a continuous half-hour amidst meetings, work tasks, and family responsibilities. As a result, they often skip meditation sessions, feeling frustrated and guilty about not meeting their goal.

Through self-awareness, they recognize that their current lifestyle does not realistically allow for a 30-minute daily meditation session. Understanding their time constraints and stress levels, they adjust their goal to meditate for just 5 minutes each day. This new goal is achievable and fits seamlessly into even the busiest of days. They can meditate during a short break, after waking up, or before going to bed.

By setting a goal that aligns with their available time and energy, they find it much easier to maintain a consistent meditation practice. The shorter duration makes it less daunting, and they experience the benefits of regular meditation, such as reduced stress and improved focus, without feeling overwhelmed. As their practice becomes a habitual part of their routine, they may gradually increase the duration as their schedule allows, but the key is starting with an achievable goal.

Example of Integration

Scenario: An individual aims to adopt a healthier lifestyle.

Everyday Participation: They decided to include a 20-minute brisk walk in their daily routine.

Simplicity Focused: They choose walking because it requires no special equipment or complex planning.

Achievable Focused: They set the goal at 20 minutes, which is realistic given their busy schedule.

Self-Aware Focused: They recognize that they enjoy morning walks, so they schedule this activity in the morning to align with their preference, ensuring consistency. They are also aware that being outdoors helps absorb vitamin D, further enhancing their health.

Purpose-Driven Aspect: They connect their daily walk to their desire to improve overall health to stay active and engaged with their family, particularly their young children.

Analysis

Consistency: The simplicity of the task ensures it's not burdensome, making daily participation likely.

Realism: The achievable nature of the goal prevents feelings of overwhelm and increases the likelihood of sticking with it.

Alignment: Self-awareness ensures that the chosen activity is enjoyable and fits well within the individual's lifestyle and needs, further supporting ongoing engagement.

Purpose: Connecting the activity to a broader life goal provides additional motivation and meaning, enhancing long-term commitment.

Conclusion

This chapter demonstrates how the principles of Simplicity Focused, Achievable Focused, and Self-Aware Focused are interconnected and collectively support the overarching principle of Everyday Participation. Each principle complements and enhances the others, creating a cohesive and sustainable approach to a healthy lifestyle. This interconnected approach ensures that health-promoting behaviors are integrated seamlessly into daily life, making a healthy lifestyle both attainable and enduring.

By understanding and embracing the interconnections between these principles and embedding a sense of purpose into your health practices, you can create a robust framework for a healthy lifestyle that is both practical and sustainable. This holistic approach not only supports your physical health but also enhances your mental and emotional well-being, paving the way for a balanced and fulfilling life. When your daily actions are driven by purpose, they become more than habits—they become meaningful steps towards a life of vitality and fulfillment.

Chapter 5

LIFESTYLE, CONSISTENCY, AND EVERYDAY PARTICIPATION

The Power of Lifestyle Choices

In the pursuit of a sustainable, healthy lifestyle, understanding the impact of our daily choices is essential. It's widely recognized that up to 90% of all diseases are related to lifestyle choices. This perspective underscores the significant influence of our everyday habits on our overall health. The food we consume, the level of physical activity we engage in, and the toxins we expose ourselves to are all critical factors that shape our well-being. While genetics provide the foundation, our lifestyle brings this blueprint to life—genetics may load the gun, but lifestyle pulls the trigger.

Consider your body as a house and your health practices as the tools needed to maintain and improve this house. Just like a physical house, your body requires regular upkeep to preserve its condition and enhance its value. Neglecting basic maintenance tasks—like cleaning the gutters or fixing leaks—can lead to significant problems later, which could be costly or even impossible to fix. Similarly, neglecting your health can lead to severe issues that require extensive medical intervention.

Maintaining your house involves routine tasks that preserve its current state while investing in it involves enhancements that increase its value. In terms of health, this translates to daily habits like proper nutrition, regular exercise, and adequate sleep (maintenance) as well as more specific practices like advanced training routines, dietary supplements, or preventive health check-ups (investment). By consistently maintaining and occasionally investing in your health, you ensure its long-term well-being and resilience.

Movement: The Catalyst for Energy

Newton's Law of Motion, which states that a body at rest will remain at rest and a body in motion will stay in motion, applies to human behavior and psychology as well. The less we move, the less we feel like moving. Conversely, the more we move, the more our bodies crave movement. Energy feeds off energy. This concept highlights the importance of integrating regular physical activity into our lives, emphasizing simplicity and achievability. Even a small commitment to daily exercise can yield significant benefits. For instance, a base-level commitment of a 15-minute workout every day may seem inconsequential, but it's far better than no workout at all. These small wins compound over time, leading to substantial improvements in health and fitness. By focusing on simple and achievable exercise routines, we can create momentum—each step forward makes the next one easier. This approach aligns with the principle of being achievable-focused, setting realistic goals that foster long-term success.

Consistency Over Perfection

Our entire lives can change with six months of consistency. It's not about being perfect every single day, but about being better than we were yesterday. Consistency trumps perfectionism because sustainable habits lead to lasting results. By focusing on gradual improvements, we build a foundation of healthy behaviors that can withstand the test of time. Getting fit is an investment in ourselves. The food we eat, the exercise we do, and the sleep we get are all daily investments in our health. These small, consistent actions lead to big dividends over time. It's like a savings account; regular deposits grow into substantial wealth. Similarly, regular healthy choices accumulate into a robust and resilient body. This principle of consistency aligns with the achievable-focused mindset, emphasizing the power of small, consistent actions.

Individual Uniqueness

Just as every house has a distinct design and set of needs, each person's body is unique, requiring personalized care and attention. This uniqueness means that what works for one person may not work for another, necessitating a tailored approach to health and wellness. Understanding and honoring your body's specific needs is crucial. Pay attention to

46

physiological and emotional cues, such as how different foods affect your energy levels, mood, and overall health. For instance, some people feel energized and clear-headed after eating lean meats, while others may experience digestive discomfort or skin issues. Processed foods often lead to sluggishness and mental fog, whereas whole, unprocessed foods promote vitality and clarity.

Tailoring your health practices involves experimenting with different foods and routines to determine what works best for you. This requires patience and self-awareness. In social settings, maintaining your personalized health plan necessitates mental strength and discipline. Set clear intentions, make mindful decisions, and choose healthier alternatives when possible or learn to moderate poor alternatives when those moments arise. By staying true to the foods and practices that make you feel healthy, energized, and satisfied, you create a sustainable, personalized health plan that supports your unique needs and overall well-being.

Prioritization of Health Aspects

Just as certain parts of a house—like the foundation, roof, and plumbing—are more critical than others, some aspects of your health require more attention. The health of your brain, gut, and kidneys, for example, should be prioritized because they play foundational roles in your overall well-being. Addressing these primary areas can indirectly support other aspects of your health, much like maintaining the foundation of a house supports its overall structure. On the other hand, issues like hair loss, while important, are secondary and often benefit from the overall improvement of your foundational health.

Flexibility in Health

Health is not a one-size-fits-all concept; it requires flexibility. Your toolbox should be equipped to handle a variety of tasks, and you need to be prepared to adapt your approach as your needs change. This flexibility is crucial because life is unpredictable, and your health needs can shift over time due to factors like aging, lifestyle changes, or new health conditions.

Everyday Participation is the Way

"Everyday Participation" is the cornerstone of effective health maintenance and improvement. The Kaizen philosophy, which emphasizes continuous incremental improvement, aligns perfectly with this idea. By focusing on "Everyday Participation," you can make small, sustainable changes that add up over time. This approach makes it easier to integrate new health practices into your daily routine without feeling overwhelmed. Combined with optimization tactics, the benefits of these integrated health practices are significantly enhanced.

Practical Tools and Strategies

There are numerous tools and strategies available to enhance and maintain your health, including a variety of diets such as the Mediterranean, ketogenic, or vegetarian diets; diverse exercise routines like strength training, calisthenics, cardio, or yoga; and various mental conditioning techniques like meditation, mindfulness, or cognitive-behavioral therapy. The key to success lies in exploring and identifying what works best for you and then optimizing that tool based on your individual capacity and needs. Often, the challenge isn't the specific diet, exercise routine, or mental conditioning technique itself. Rather, it is about tailoring each approach to fit your unique circumstances and capabilities. By aligning health practices with your personal capacity, you can maximize their effectiveness and sustainability.

Preventive Health Care

One of the most critical aspects of maintaining your health is prevention. Don't wait until problems become severe. Early intervention is often simpler and more effective. Regular check-ups, a balanced diet that focuses on whole foods rather than processed foods, and an active lifestyle can prevent many health issues from developing in the first place. From that starting point, you can move forward in making adjustments that align with your body, your mind, and your soul.

Health System Limitations

Our current health systems are primarily designed to manage diseases rather than prevent them. This management approach often leads to a reactive rather than proactive mindset. Unfortunately, there are few profitable business models focused on curing or preventing health problems, as the medical industry often profits more from treating chronic conditions. Therefore, it's essential to take personal responsibility for your health. Educate yourself, make informed decisions, and prioritize preventive care to avoid becoming a victim of a system that may not always have your best interests at heart.

Taking Personal Responsibility

Ultimately, the responsibility for maintaining and improving your health lies with you. Equip yourself with the knowledge and tools needed to take care of your body. By doing so, you can avoid many of the pitfalls associated with neglect and ensure that you live a healthier, more fulfilling life. That is true empowerment.

Conclusion

In this chapter, we have explored the profound impact of lifestyle consistency and the principles of Everyday Participation. The journey towards optimal health is not about extreme measures or quick fixes but about making informed, sustainable choices that integrate seamlessly into your daily life. By focusing on small, achievable actions that align with your personal goals and capacities, you can build a foundation for lasting health and well-being.

Remember, your health is a dynamic and evolving aspect of your life, influenced by a myriad of factors, including diet, physical activity, and mental conditioning. The strategies and tools discussed, from various diets and exercise routines to mental health techniques, are all valuable resources. However, their true power lies in how well they are tailored to your individual needs and circumstances.

Consistency, simplicity, and self-awareness are the cornerstones of this approach. By simplifying your health practices, setting realistic goals, and cultivating a deep understanding of your own needs, you can create a sustainable and fulfilling health journey. This method ensures that each small step you take is purposeful and aligned with your broader life goals, making the path to health both manageable and meaningful.

Ultimately, embracing the principles of Everyday Participation allows you to transform your daily habits into powerful tools for well-being. Each action, no matter how small, contributes to your overall health and resilience, leading to a more vibrant and fulfilling life. As you continue to implement these strategies, remember that the journey is as important as the destination. Celebrate your progress, learn from your challenges, and stay committed to your goals. Your dedication to a healthier lifestyle is an investment in yourself that will pay dividends in every aspect of your life.

Conclusion

OPTIMIZING YOUR LIFESTYLE FOR THE GREATEST RETURN ON INVESTMENT

As we draw this journey of "Everyday Participation" to a close, it's crucial to acknowledge the importance of sustainable and manageable health practices. Just as achieving a 100% return on investment (ROI) daily is virtually unattainable in the financial world, so too is expecting extraordinary returns from extreme health efforts. The greater the investment relative to your capacity, the riskier it becomes to sustain. This understanding is vital in making informed decisions tailored to individual circumstances.

For instance, a daily 0.25% ROI on a $100,000 investment significantly impacts someone earning $35,000 annually but is negligible to a billionaire. This example illustrates that the threshold of meaningful returns varies for each person. Similarly, in health and wellness, understanding your capacity and limits for physical activity, mindfulness, and diet is crucial. Knowing your threshold for maintaining consistent participation in healthy practices is essential.

Engaging in manageable, simple, and meaningful health behaviors consistently allows these actions to become habitual.

Over time, habitual engagement in healthy practices increases resilience to poor health choices and enhances the ability to make decisions without mental distress. This approach ensures that you can sustain a healthier lifestyle with greater ease and confidence.

By focusing on the principles of Simplicity Focused, Achievable Focused, and Self-Aware Focused, "Everyday Participation" offers a holistic approach that emphasizes the importance of personal context. These principles form the cornerstone of a proactive approach to health and well-being, empowering you to integrate healthy habits into your daily life effectively.

The Power of Oxytocin

One often overlooked aspect of optimizing health is the role of oxytocin, commonly known as the "love hormone." Oxytocin plays a vital role in fostering social bonds, reducing stress, and enhancing overall well-being. Understanding how to increase and maintain high levels of oxytocin can be transformative, particularly during times of stress and challenge.

Oxytocin not only fosters a sense of connection and trust but also helps mitigate the effects of cortisol, the stress hormone. When stress levels rise and life feels overwhelming, our bodies produce more cortisol, which can negatively impact our ability to function well and make healthy decisions. Elevated cortisol levels are associated with increased cravings for unhealthy foods, reduced motivation to exercise, and difficulty maintaining a positive outlook. By contrast, oxytocin promotes relaxation and reduces anxiety, making it easier to engage in and sustain healthy behaviors.

Engaging in activities that boost oxytocin levels strengthens our connection with others and ourselves, fostering a supportive environment that encourages better health choices. When oxytocin levels are high, we are more likely to feel motivated to participate in healthy activities, stick to nutritious diets, and maintain regular physical activity. This hormone's positive influence on mood and stress resilience creates a feedback loop where healthy behaviors become more rewarding and easier to maintain.

Activities to Increase Oxytocin Levels

- **Physical Touch:** Hugging, massages, holding hands, and cuddling with a partner, family member, or pet.
- **Social Interactions:** Spending time with loved ones, socializing, and participating in group activities like team sports or group exercises.
- **Acts of Kindness:** Helping others, volunteering, and giving sincere compliments.
- **Mindfulness and Relaxation:** Meditation, deep breathing exercises, and relaxation techniques.

- **Recreational Activities:** Dancing, listening to music, and sharing laughter.
- **Pet Interaction:** Playing with, petting, or simply being around pets.
- **Romantic Activities:** Kissing and sexual activity.

Incorporating these activities into your daily routine aligns perfectly with the principles of Everyday Participation, Simplicity Focused, Achievable Focused, and Self-Aware Focused. These activities are simple, sustainable, and deeply personal, making them easy to integrate into your life. By prioritizing oxytocin-boosting activities, you create a supportive foundation for maintaining consistent and positive health practices.

Optimizing Your Lifestyle

Optimizing your lifestyle isn't solely about longevity; it's about enhancing every moment of your life. When you simplify your choices, set achievable goals, and align your actions with your personal needs, you provide yourself with the foundation for a balanced and fulfilling existence. This approach ensures that each day is lived to the fullest, with vitality and purpose guiding your path.

Remember, optimizing your lifestyle is a journey, not a destination. Embrace the process of growth and self-improvement, celebrate milestones along the way, and learn from setbacks with resilience and determination. Every positive choice you make contributes to a healthier, more vibrant you, enhancing your overall quality of life and enriching the lives of those around you.

FAREWELL

As you embark on this journey of optimizing your lifestyle through Everyday Participation, guided by Simplicity Focused, Achievable Focused, and Self-Aware Focused principles, know that you hold the brush to create a masterpiece of health and happiness. By investing in yourself today, you sow the seeds for a future filled with vitality, purpose, and boundless possibilities. Your life is your canvas—paint it with intention, nurture it with care, and watch as each stroke enhances the masterpiece that is your quality of life.

Call-To-Action

EVERYDAY PARTICIPATION ASSESSMENT FORM

Ready to transform your life FOREVER? Take the first step today by filling out my Everyday Participation Assessment Form! Discover how to simplify your habits, set achievable goals, and enhance self-awareness on your journey to a healthier, more fulfilling life.

After completing the form, connect with me personally. Together, we'll tailor personalized recommendations that promote simplicity, achievability, and self-awareness, ensuring your path to everyday participation in a vibrant life. Let's embark on this transformative journey together!

https://owlgoodinvestments.com/epassessmentform

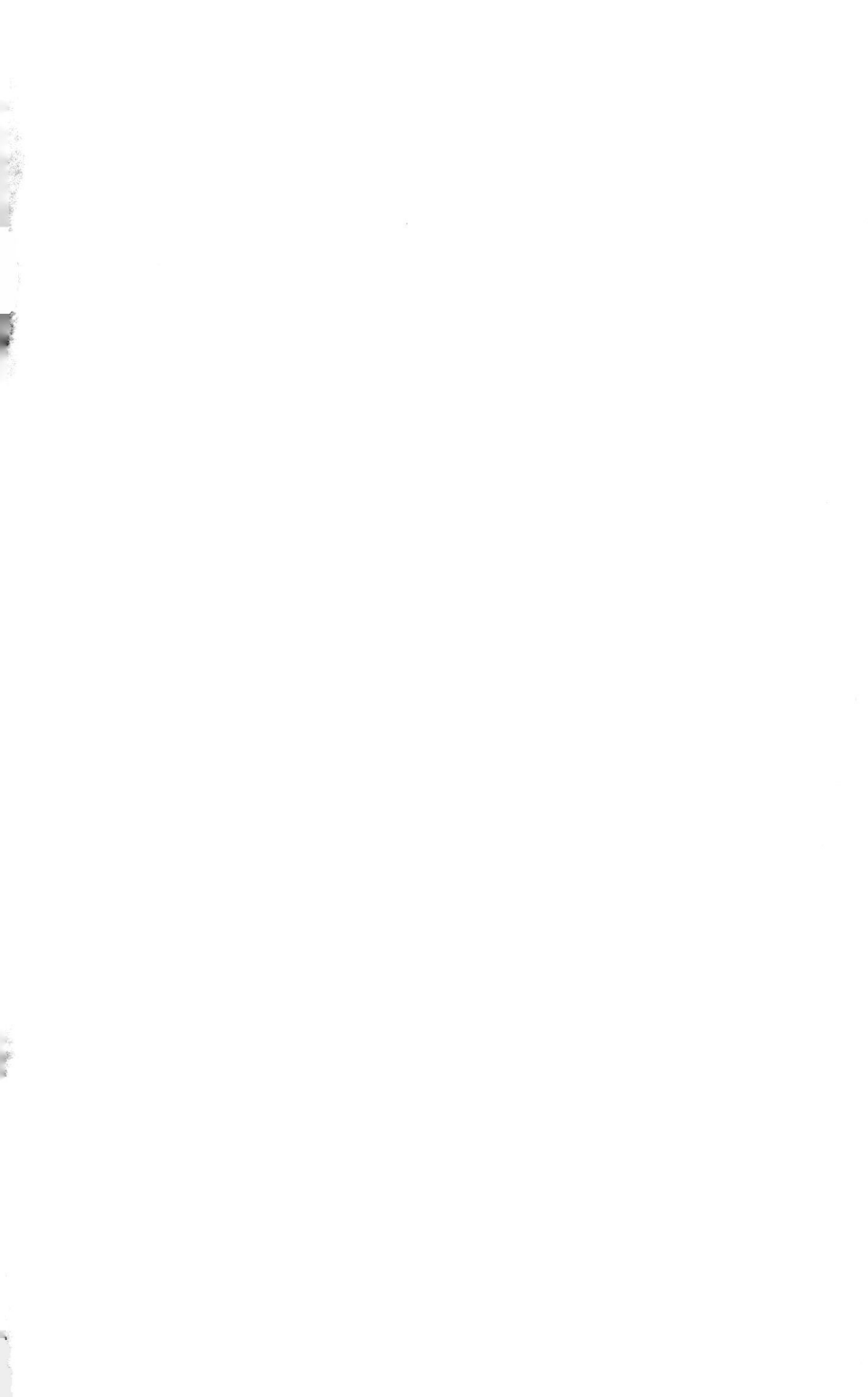

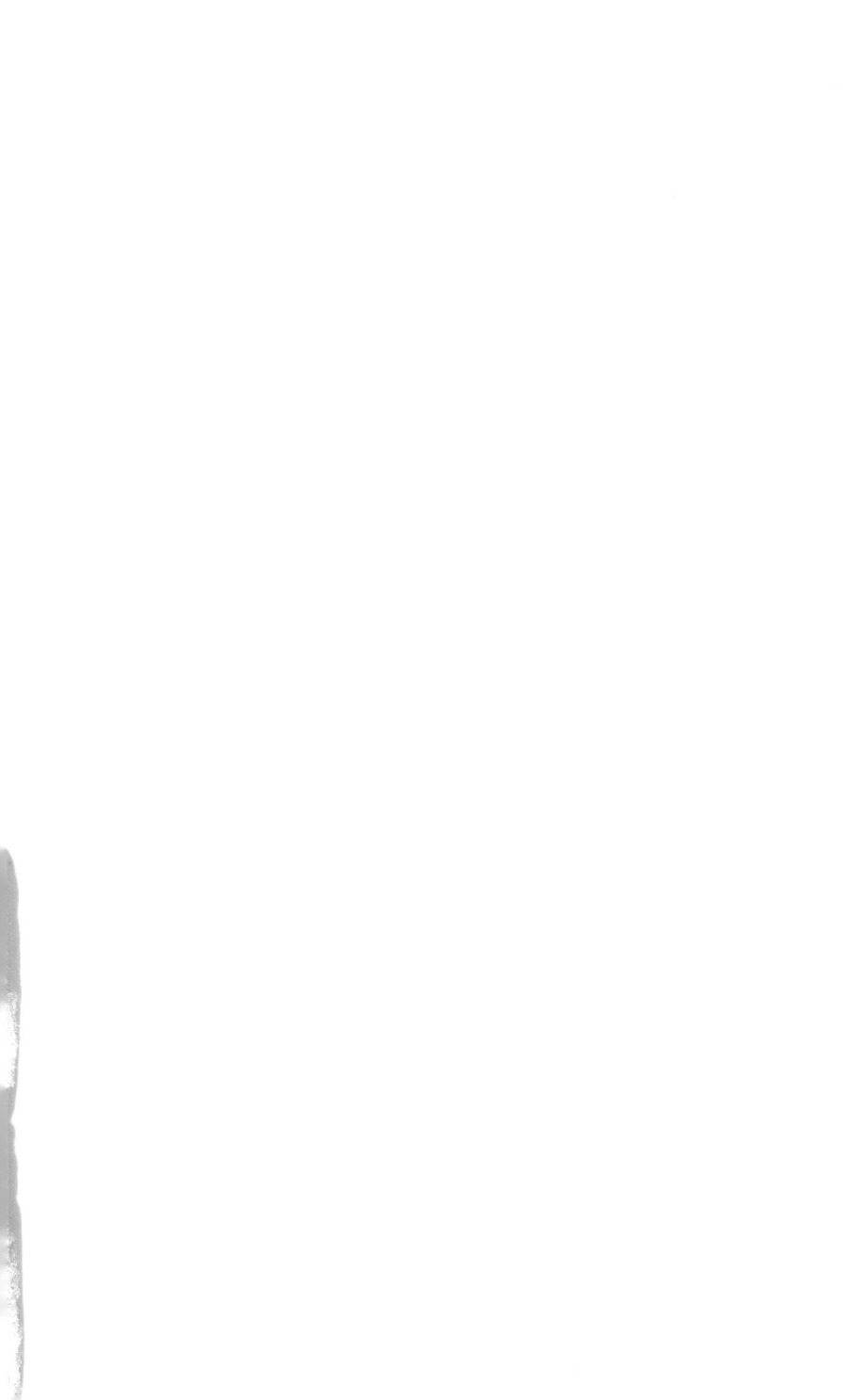